KILLING SOAP

KILLING SOAP

STOP POLLUTING YOURSELF AND OUR WATER

Richard Tieken

Copyright © 2016 Richard Tieken

ISBN-10: 1539770443
EAN-13: 9781539770442

I AM WRITING THIS BOOK TO EXPLAIN TO THE READER HOW I CAME TO THE CONCLUSION THAT I HAVE BEEN DOING SOMETHING IMPROPER ALL MY LIFE AND AT MY AGE OF 83 YEARS I WANT TO SHARE THIS EXPERIENCE. YES, IT HAS TO DO WITH BATHING. I WILL BRING YOU ALONG THROUGH MY EXPERIENCES GRADUALLY LEADING TO THE FINAL CONCLUSION.

About 1945 I was sitting in a history class at Shenandoah Junior High School in Miami, Florida. I am a day dreamer and not all that interested in the subject matter. A person came into the class room with an announcement that the dining room kitchen needed some help right now and was anyone interested? I jumped up and said YES. The pay was $3.00 a week and the work was washing trays during the lunch hour so it would not interfere with my classes. They wanted me now so they could train me on how to run the tray washing machine.

It was not difficult to learn and I got right to it, picking up speed as I went along. Steam from the hot soapy water was pouring out of the machine and I was told to make sure the water stayed as hot as it was so the soap scum was melted off the trays. If the trays came out all spotless, shiny and clean looking they should be safe to eat from. I was also told that if the water was not 180 degrees then soap scum would remain on the trays and collect bacteria which would immediately contaminate any food placed on the tray. The lady who ran the lunch room would go around inspecting the washing of dishes and food preparation and serving. I was really impressed with the efficiency of this operation on top of the $3.00 a week which I saved in my dresser drawer at home.

In 1953 I went to ROTC Summer Camp at Fort Benning, Georgia while a student at Gordon Military College in Barnesville, Georgia. I was put on KP duty (kitchen police) for one day and since I was already an experienced tray washer I volunteered for that work. I must have washed over 200 trays when the Mess Sergeant came buy, examined the trays and said I had to wash them all over again. He checked the water temperature and it was not hot enough and he showed me the soap scum on the trays.

He did not get mad at me even though I felt guilty because I should have known. The water was steaming but the temperature was just not sufficiently hot. Fortunately none of these trays had been put out for use so no one got sick.

I know that what I have so far written is nothing really new to the reader. Our home dish washers recommend we use 180 degree hot water though

KILLING SOAP

maybe they don't explain why. So now let's get to our daily showering where we use a bar of soap and a wash cloth. How refreshing this is and how very clean we feel after we dry off and slip into those nice clean clothes to begin our day. Well, I went into the Army in 1956 to my chosen branch Infantry. I was a Captain when I volunteered for Adviser Duty in Vietnam in 1965. I went through the six weeks training at Fort Bragg, North Carolina where we learned more about the war, what to expect and about the different terrain in that country as we would have to select the part of Vietnam we wanted to be assigned to. The Delta in the South (low land, canals and not many trees), jungle in the middle and mountains in the North. Of course there was the long coast line which made up the eastern part of South Vietnam and North Vietnam. I selected the middle part. An American Colonel was the Senior Division Adviser and if you wanted to be one of the Vietnamese Infantry Battalion Advisers then you had to tell the Colonel that is what you wanted. It was a very dangerous job as you went where your battalion went and assisted them with air strikes, medical evacuations and fighting alongside them. I asked for this job for professional reasons. I had, as part of my team, a lieutenant, a senior NCO and a radio operator. I also had a Vietnamese soldier for a jeep driver.

RICHARD TIEKEN

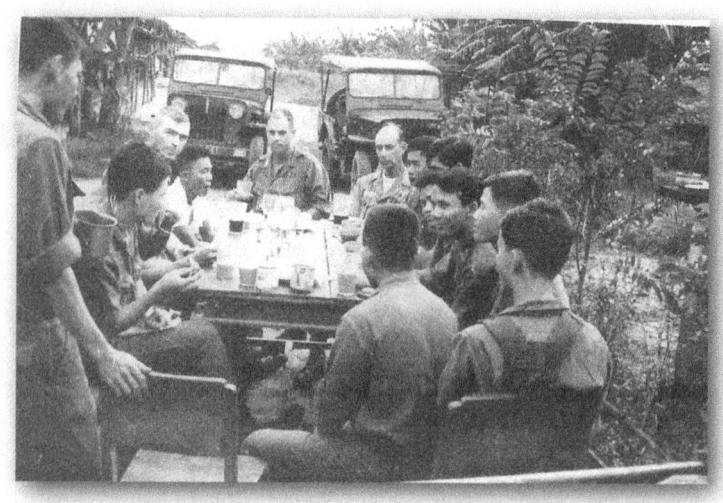

Officers of the 1st Battalion 7th Regiment 5th ARVN
Richard Tieken (Head of the table)

KILLING SOAP

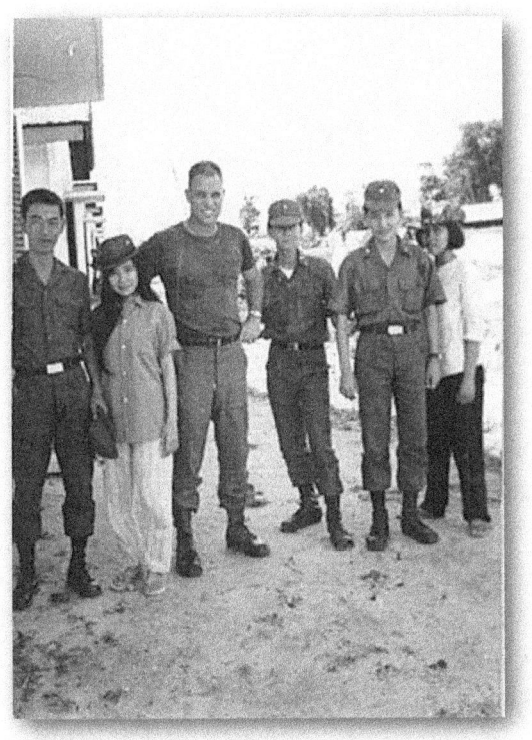

Psyops girls me with my interperter_VN 1965

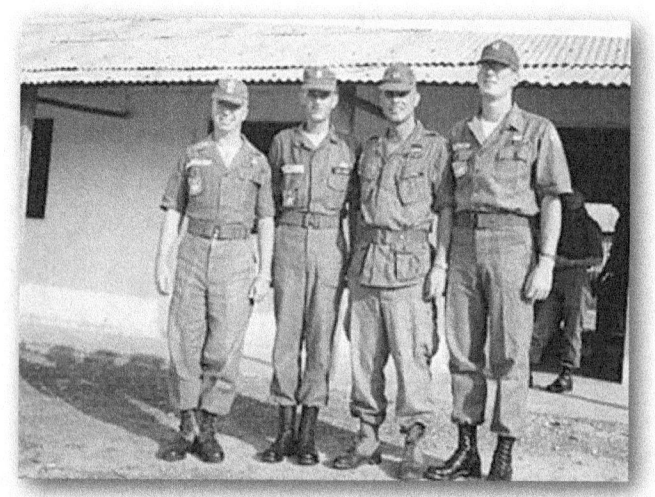

Bn Advisor's 7th Regt Capt's De Leuil Hinds Tieken Sparling

You are probably wondering by now just what does all this have to do with the subject of this book?

Well, I have gotten to that. When you are in the jungle for long periods of time, your nose becomes more sensitive because you are not around industrial or people made pollution. The Vietnamese would tell me that the enemy (Viet Cong) could smell an American Unit a mile away. At the time I did not pay any attention to these statements only maybe it was because we used shaving lotion and smoked cigarettes. Early in the war this may have been true but those habits were quickly stopped. I took my usual showers when we were in our small base camps but when we went out on operations there were Vietnamese soldiers detailed to provide a bathing facility. This consisted of three soldiers holding up ponchos for your privacy while another soldier poured a small pale of water over your head and gave you another pale of water to splash on other parts of your body. One then gave you a small towel to dry off with. I think they did this for only the higher ranked personnel letting the others take care of themselves. I felt sort of stupid going through every day on combat and reconnaissance operations.

One day in a village I noticed a rain barrel in the center of a house where rain water was diverted through a hole into the roof into the rain barrel. I gradually realized that this is how the people bathed as I was offered this chance a few times and took advantage of the situation. No one used soap! You just took your clothes off and with a pale you dipped it in the rain barrel and then poured the water directly on top of your head. There was a place next to the water container where you stood and the water you poured over your head and on your body just ran off into the ground. No problem. It only took two pales of water and some just used one pale. The rain barrels stayed full during the rainy season. During the dry season a big water truck would go through the villages filling up the water barrels. At this point I want to say one important thing, these people did not have offensive body odor which we at times do. They always smelled clean and I could not

KILLING SOAP

understand why. I lived with the Vietnamese for one year so I know what I am talking about.

In 2015 I was reading the February issue of Popular Mechanics magazine. In there was an article on washing your hands without using soap. They said that if you are in a crowed restroom and need to wash your hands then just get some water on your hands and clean them that way. What happens is that water breaks the protective cell around the bacteria and thus kills it. Soap will not do this. Now I am starting to put two and two together and coming to the conclusion that this must also happen when you take a shower. I noticed that after three days using my same wash cloth it started to stink. That is the soap scum staying on the wash cloth and giving a nice home to multiples of bacteria. I tried the same thing using a wash cloth but no soap. After three days the wash cloth still smelled as clean as if it were new.

The above is a test you can do yourself. The proof that using soap when you take a bath or shower harbors the bacteria that makes you smell bad is right there. In the meantime I also discovered that the Vietnamese people do not use soap in their bathing, only clear water. While I was in

Vietnam the US Government (USAID) was giving out bars of soap to the Vietnamese people obviously in the hope of getting them to use it on a regular basis. I would imagine that what little money these people had, especially in the villages, they could buy a week's supply of rice for the price of a bar of soap. But even in the cities and hotels where the locals had showers, THE PEOPLE DID NOT USE SOAP.

I took showers with the Vietnamese officers and noticed that they did not use soap. Now I know why. It is a stupid habit that has been with us for hundreds of years. What is soap? It is animal fat and this stuff harbors bacteria like no one's business. I was riding around on the edge of the Florida Everglades one time and I smelled this terrible odor. I asked the older gentleman I was riding with what that odor was and he replied that it was a soap factory. Boy, did it stink. I bet you could easily smell it two miles down wind.

I have gone almost one year now without using soap when I shower and I am cleaner and smell better in all parts of my body than I have in previous years. I will never go back to using soap in my shower. I do use a wash cloth to get to those hard to get

KILLING SOAP

places and this works well, I just don't put any soap on the wash cloth. It stays clean smelling.

You can go online and look up, "bathing without soap" and you will see some tests that were conducted on men, women and children with amazing results. Why this news doesn't get out, I don't know. I have discussed this subject with my Army Fort Benning Dermatologist and she seemed very favorable when I discussed this subject with her as well as another dermatologist that worked with her. I have contacted interested personnel in the Department of Army and also The Center for Disease Control. I have not heard back from them as of the time of this writing but I also did not ask for any feedback.

Millions of people wash almost daily with soap. They are contaminating their skin with soap scum that they cannot completely wash off so they add a nice home for bacteria to thrive. The longer it stays on your skin the more it stinks, especially in those tight areas like under your arms. That is why under arm deodorant is so widely used. I have not used any since I stopped using soap and I do admit that I still get a bit of odor from under my arms but water takes the odor away for some hours. Think of all the soap (animal fat) that gets into our water supply every minute of every day when it washes down the drain. Literally tons of it, all over the world. This has to build up into the ground.

I read about aircraft carrier operations in the Pacific during World War II and one article I read was a concern from one of the medical doctors. He said that pilots should shower every day so that in the event they get wounded their wounds won't be so badly contaminated. No one realized at that time that the contamination was mostly caused by the soap scum bacteria. The longer you went without bathing than the greater buildup of bacteria so when you received an open wound, healing became a problem. By the time you got back to your carrier and received medical attention for your wounds, the bacteria had already gotten a head start.

There would be a tremendous advantage if military units would stop using soap in bathing (1) it would require less water in the field, (2) the soldiers would smell better (3) it would be one less item the units would have to supply (4) wounded soldiers would heal faster (6) shower stalls in barracks would stay cleaner. For submarine crews, I think it would be very advantages because of the close quarters

KILLING SOAP

they are living in and the absence of soapy water to dispose of. I have never served on a submarine but I can use a little common sense here.

I want to finish up with water contamination. We hear so much these days about how the future will be for the supply of clean water for the people masses. The population of the earth is increasing at a very rapid rate so I can understand the concern. I would think that getting people to stop bathing with soap will pay off in big dividends in the future as well as the present. It is a difficult thing to convince people to change their bathing habits to what I am suggesting here. I have tried with some friends of mine and about half go for it and the other half don't even want to try it. You can take the wash cloth test like I suggested earlier and that should be positive proof for anyone.

I went online (Wikipedia) to see what other sources of information were available on this subject and I came up with some following interesting facts:

1. Almost all bacteria are invisible to the naked dye.
2. Bacteria can double every 20 minutes under ideal conditions.

3. Bacteria are surrounded by a cell wall which give them protection. Water will break that cell wall thus killing the bacteria.
4. There are instances of soap being made from human body fat. There is evidence from the Nuremberg Trials that Germans had found a way to do this.

HOW DOES SOAP WORK

Soap allows dirt on our bodies to become soluble in water so it can be rinsed away. Water alone will wash away the dirt and perspiration from our skin but if you worked in a coal mine and your skin was covered with coal dust and dirt then water alone would not do a thorough cleaning job. Soap would allow the dirt to become soluble in water where it would easily wash away. When you use soap to clean your skin then you need 170 degree hot water to remove all of the soap scum and kill the bacteria. Our skin cannot tolerate water at this high temperature so you leave the shower with sufficient soap still on your skin to harbor bacteria and at the warm temperature of your body, especially in the hard to get to places like under your arms, the bacteria can double every 20 MINUTES. This naturally creates body odor.

ANIMAL FAT

I was worried that reducing the amount of soap made from animal fat would create a problem by causing an oversupply of fat that would somehow have to be gotten rid of. I went online and found out that it should not be a problem. The large meat company Tyson Foods has invested with another company, Syntroleum Corporation who are testing ways for converting low-grade inedible fats and greases into a renewable diesel fuel for transportation.

Scientists have been looking for raw materials that can be made into a fuel-source that doesn't divert food into energy and is abundant enough that can make a significant dent into the oil market. I guess a person can then summarize that by reducing the amount of soap we use at home will free up more animal fat for more valuable and newer uses. I still keep soap on my bathroom sink as I wash my hands several times a day because I work on vehicles and in my yard where they get very dirty.

I don't know how long it takes the soap scum left on your body to eventually wash off. I would think at least a month. Tests that were done on people were conducted after they hadn't used it for six months.

Maybe this is a good guide to go on. I would keep on shampooing your hair in your usual manner.

ANTIBACTERIAL SOAPS

The Food and Drug Administration orders antibacterials removed from soaps. Companies will have a year to take the ingredients, triclosan and trilocarban, out of the products because they did not document that the ingredients were both safe for long term daily use and did nothing to kill germs.

ABOUT THE AUTHOR

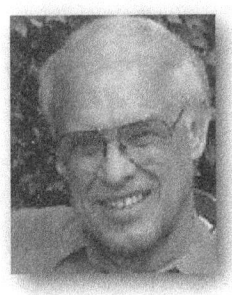

RICHARD V. TIEKEN was born in Peoria, Illinois but grew up in Louisville, Kentucky and later in Miami, Florida. He is a graduate of Mercer University in Macon, Georgia and served 20 years in the US Army as a combat infantry officer. His assignments included eight years in Germany, two years in Vietnam. He retired from the Army as a Major then went into the retail liquor store business owning and managing his own liquor store, Holly Hills Beverage Shop, for 32 years in Columbus, Georgia His wife, June Lee, retired from teaching Earth Science at Troy University about the same time. A little more about June, she

RICHARD TIEKEN

grew up in the British Crown Colony of Hong Kong where I met her at King George V (KGV) school. She earned a master degree in Geology from Ball State University in Muncie, Indiana and retired a professor of the sciences.

www.ingramcontent.com/pod-product-compliance
Lightning Source LLC
Chambersburg PA
CBHW070720210526
45170CB00021B/1386